Maroua Garma
Sameh Sioud
Habib Hamdi

Diagnosis and treatment of oral lichen planus

Maroua Garma
Sameh Sioud
Habib Hamdi

Diagnosis and treatment of oral lichen planus

ScienciaScripts

Imprint

Cover image: www.ingimage.com

This book is a translation from the original published under ISBN 978-613-8-42573-1.

Publisher:
Sciencia Scripts
is a trademark of
Dodo Books Indian Ocean Ltd. and OmniScriptum S.R.L publishing group

120 High Road, East Finchley, London, N2 9ED, United Kingdom
Str. Armeneasca 28/1, office 1, Chisinau MD-2012, Republic of Moldova, Europe
Printed at: see last page
ISBN: 978-620-8-25978-5

CONTENTS

INTRODUCTION 2

1.CLINICAL OBSERVATION NO. 1 3

2.CLINICAL OBSERVATION NO. 2 8

DISCUSSION 11

CONCLUSION 43

REFERENCES 44

INTRODUCTION

Lichen planus is a benign chronic inflammatory mucocutaneous dermatosis affecting the skin, skin appendages and mucous membranes, including the oral mucosa, either separately or in association with lesions of the rest of the mucous membranes. Oral lichen planus tends to affect middle-aged people, with a predilection for women. This disease is characterised by a succession of phases in which the lesions are often symmetrical and develop in flare-ups. Various pathognomonic clinical forms of oral lichen planus have been described in different regions of the oral mucosa. Although for some authors the clinical diagnosis is obvious, confirmation requires a combination of both clinical and histological features. The treatment of this dermatosis tends to be symptomatic, with the aim of stabilising the lesions in a quiescent state, and several therapies have been reported for this purpose. Despite the benign nature of the disease, malignant transformation has also been described, requiring continuous monitoring. The aim of this book is to review the clinical and histological features of oral lichen planus and detail the diagnostic and therapeutic approach, while illustrating these data from the literature with two clinical observations.

1. CLINICAL OBSERVATION NO. 1

A 78-year-old hypertensive patient undergoing treatment consulted for troublesome lesions on her lower lip and the inside of her cheeks. On exobuccal clinical examination, the lips were inhomogeneously coloured, with bullae, erosions, crusts and whitish streaks in places **(Figure 1).**

On endobuccal examination, we noted :

- Poor oral hygiene **(Figure 2).**

- Decayed and dilapidated residual teeth **(Figure 2).**

- Generalised gingival recession **(Figure 2)**

- The presence of erosive patches and bullae on the inside of the lower lip and cheeks **(Figure 3).**

- Whitish streaks on the lower lip, with a whitish network associated with erosive patches on the inside of the cheeks **(Figure 4).**

These lesions were bilateral and symmetrical.

Radiological examination using panoramic radiography showed lysis. generalised horizontal bone **(Figure 5).**

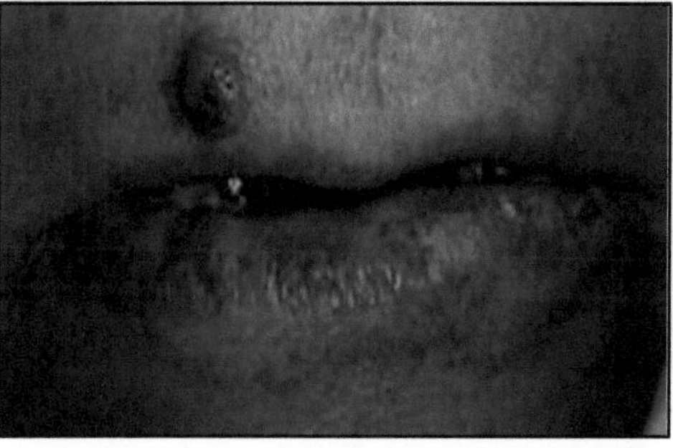

Figure 1: Presence of erosions, bullae, crusts and whitish streaks on the lower lip

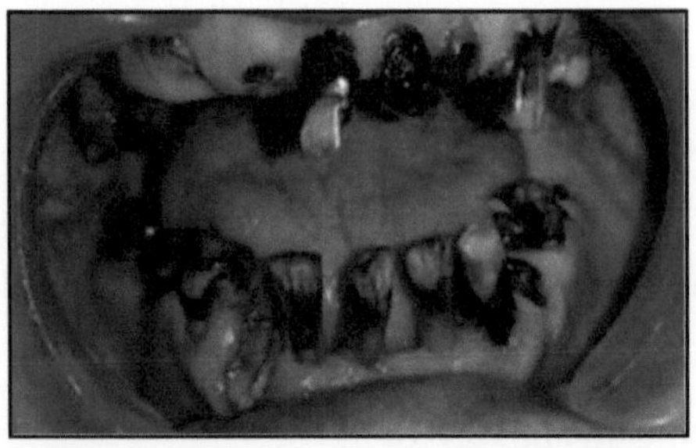

Figure 2: Generalised gingival recession with decayed and dilapidated teeth.

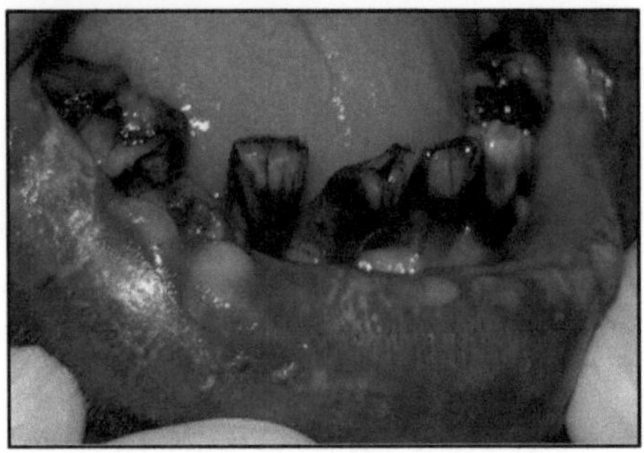

Figure 3: Erosions, bullae, crusts and whitish streaks on the inside of the lower lip.

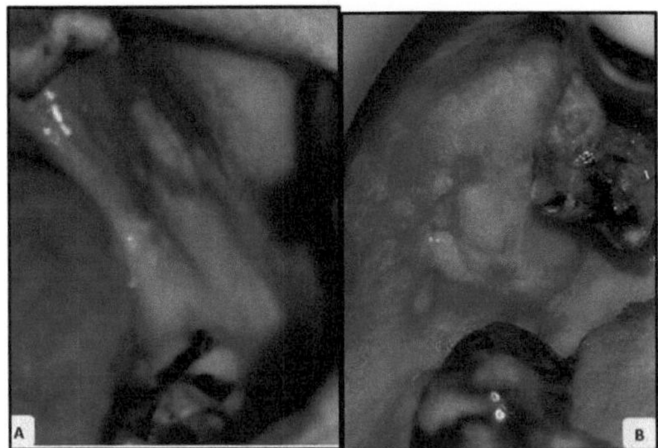

Figure 4: A-B: Bubbles associated with erosive patches with a whitish network appearance on the inside of the cheeks.

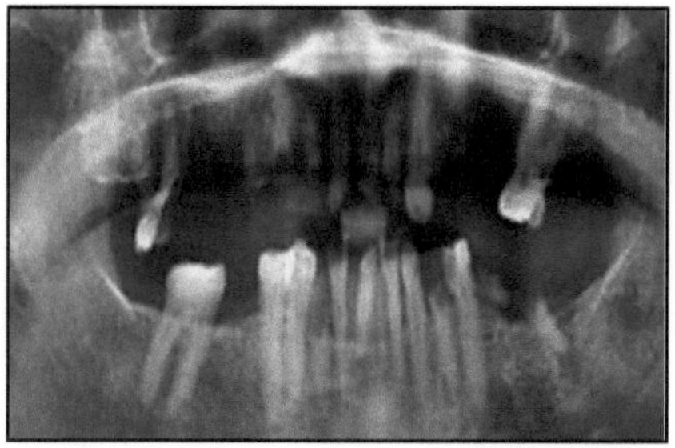

Figure 5: Panoramic radiograph showing generalised horizontal bone lysis.

The diagnosis of bullo-erosive oral lichen planus was well suspected given the presence of characteristic clinical signs:

Presence of bilateral and symmetrical lesions;

Pathognomonic whitish network appearance;

Presence of erosions and bubbles in association with this whitish network;

But diagnostic confirmation required the combination of histological criteria, and the presence of bullae meant that any other bullous disease had to be ruled out. Consequently, histological examination and direct immunofluorescence (DIF) were performed. **(Figure 6).**

IFD was negative and pathological examination confirmed the diagnosis.

suspected.

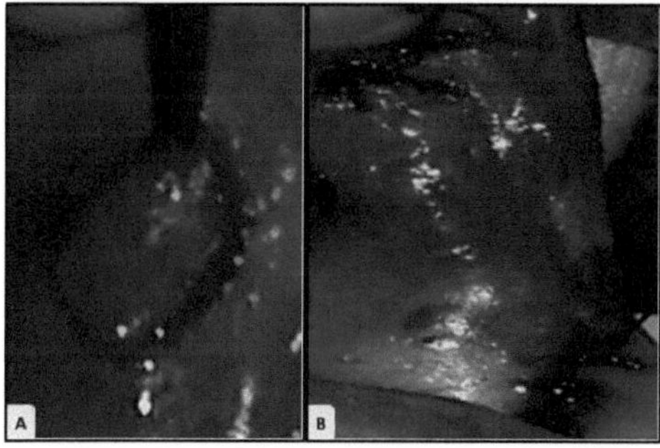

Figure 6: A-B: Biopsy for histological examination and direct immunofluorescence.

The therapeutic decision was to restore the oral cavity: extraction of all residual teeth and referral for prosthetic rehabilitation, prescription of Solupred ® (20 mg) as a mouthwash at a rate of 2 Cp*3/day and dermocorticoid: Dermocort ® to be applied to the lips three times a day. Biological tests were ordered: fasting glycaemia, hepatitis C serology and a thyroid work-up (TSH, T3, T4). All results were unremarkable.At the various follow-up sessions, progress was favourable with remission of the erosions, and the appearance of the quiescent whitish network was still present. The patient was asymptomatic and undergoing prosthetic rehabilitation. The dose of treatment was reduced as the patient progressed. **(Figure 7,8,9).**

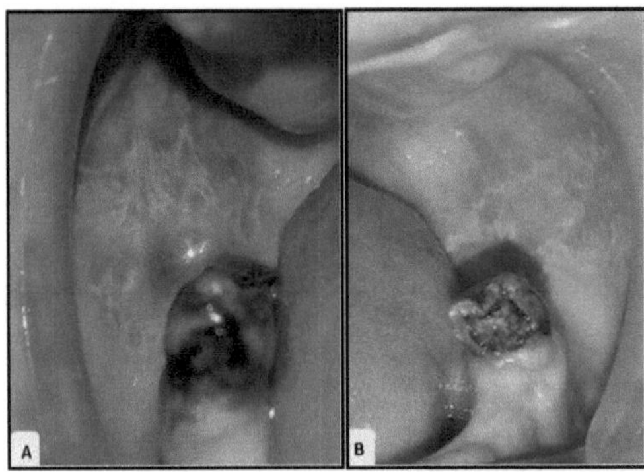

Figure 7: Favourable evolution: remission of lesions, bilateral quiescent network appearance on the inner sides of the cheeks

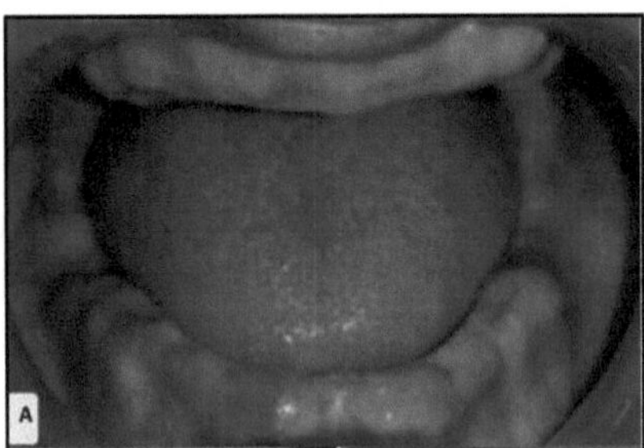

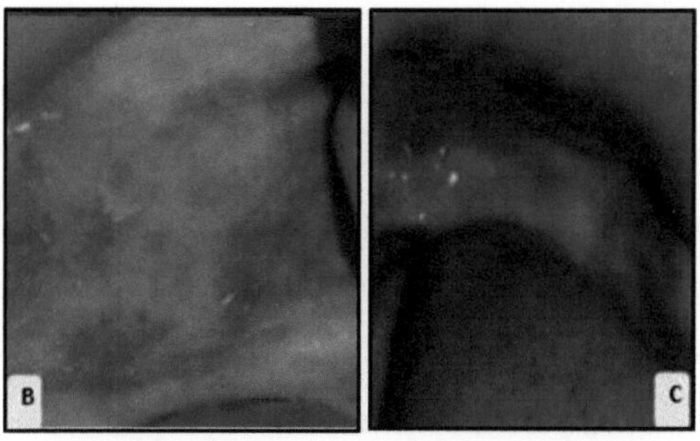

Figure 8: A, B, C: Patient with total edentulism, favourable outcome, atrophic scarring of lesions

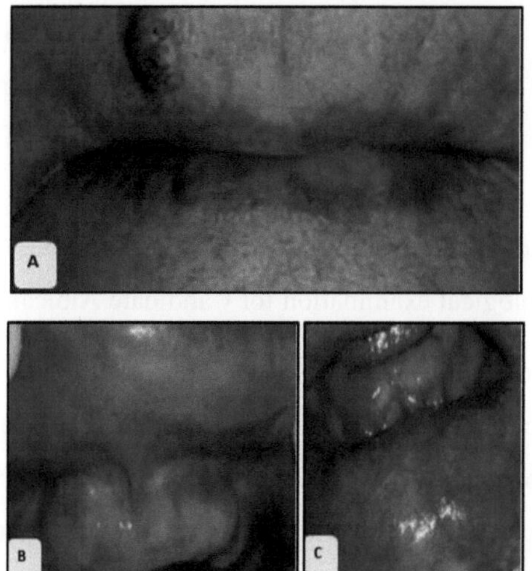

Figure 9: A, B, C: Disappearance of lesions and quiescent appearance of the lips

2. CLINICAL OBSERVATION NO. 2

A 64-year-old female patient with no notable pathological history consulted the Department of Oral Medicine and Surgery at the University Hospital Clinic of Dentistry in Monastir for a sensation of burning and tingling in the oral cavity and painful lesions on the inside of the cheeks. On exobuccal clinical examination, the lower part of the face is collapsed, the mucosa lip was atrophic.Endobuccally, the patient was totally edentulous. On the inner surfaces of the cheeks, erosions and bullae associated with whitish striae arranged in a meshwork pattern were observed. The lesions were bilateral and symmetrical. The rest of the oral mucosa was normal except for simple atrophy **(Figure 10).**
The diagnosis of oral lichen planus superinfected with candidiasis was suspected.
A biopsy for histological examination and direct immunofluorescence were performed. A mycological examination for Candidate Albicans was requested.

Anatomopathological examination confirmed the diagnosis of bullo-erosive oral lichen planus. Mycological examination was negative. The course of action was to prescribe a local corticosteroid: Solupred® 20 mg, 2 Cp*3/day. Biological tests were ordered: fasting glycaemia, thyroid work-up, hepatitis C serology.
Fasting blood glucose and thyroid function tests were normal, but hepatitis C serology was positive. The patient was then referred to the gastrology department for further investigation and was declared cured after genotyping, which did not detect HCV RNA, and viral load testing, which was also undetectable. **(Figure 11).**
The follow-up sessions were reassuring, and progress was favourable under treatment. **(Figures 12 and 13).**

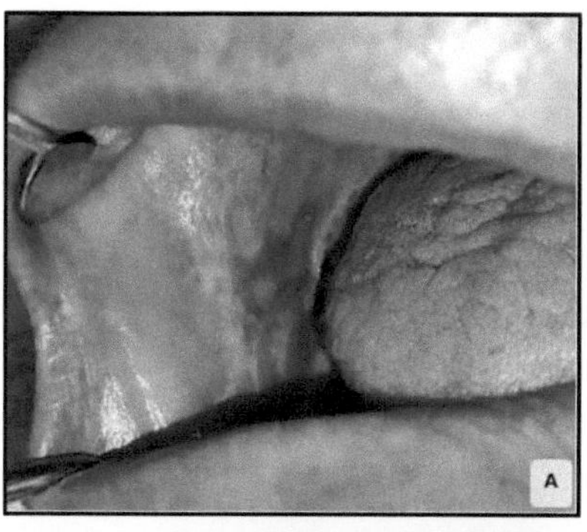

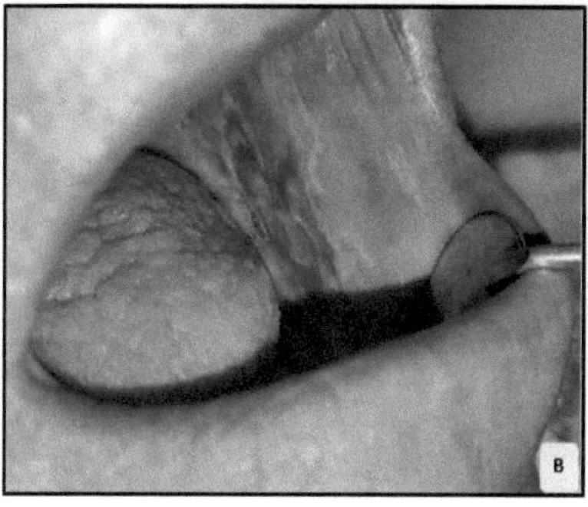

Figure 10: A/B: Erosions and bullae associated with a whitish network on the inside of the cheeks

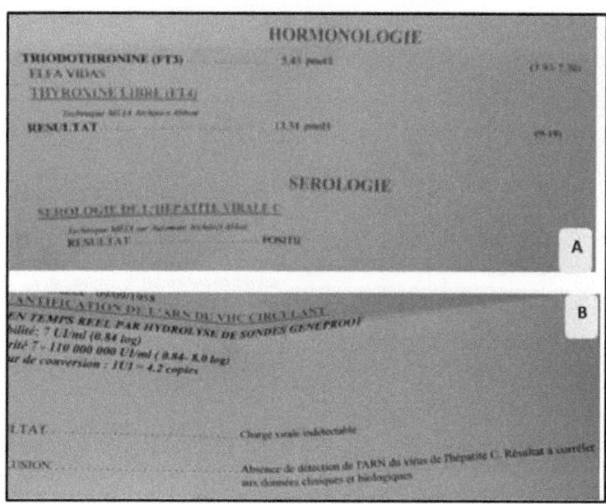

HORMONOLOGIE

TRIODOTHRONINE (FT3)

THYROXINE LIBRE (FT4)

RESULTAT

SEROLOGIE

RESULTAT .... POSITIF

A

...ANTIFICATION DE L'ARN DU VHC CIRCULANT

...EN TEMPS REEL PAR HYDROLYSE DE SONDES GENEPROOF

...bilité: 7 UI/ml (0.84 log)

...rité 7 - 110 000 000 UI/ml (0.84- 8.0 log)

...ur de conversion : 1UI = 4.2 copies

B

...LTAT .... Charge virale indétectable

...USION .... Absence de détection de l'ARN du virus de l'hépatite C. Résultat à corréler aux données cliniques et biologiques

Figure 11: Hepatitis C serology, viral load detection and genotyping

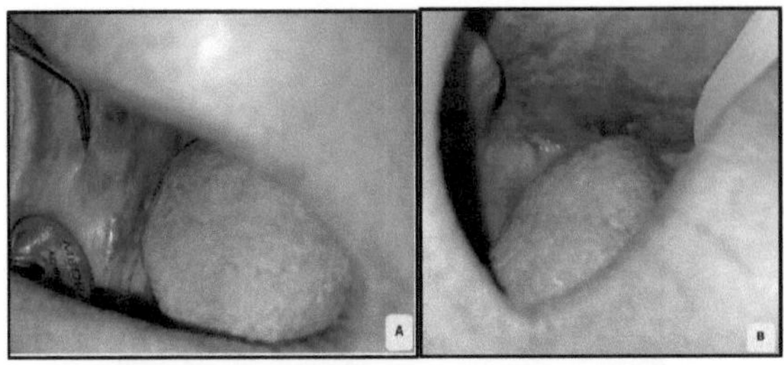

Figure 12: A/B: Favourable evolution, lesions begin to regress

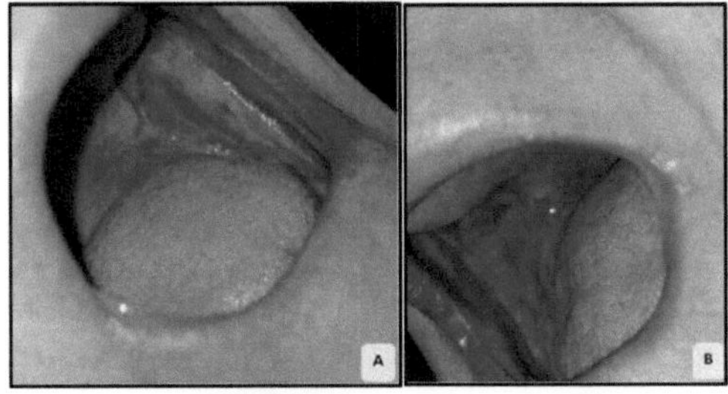

Figure 13: A/B: Very favourable evolution, Quescent whitish network appearance

DISCUSSION

1. Definition

Lichen planus (LP) is a benign chronic inflammatory mucocutaneous disease whose aetiology is still poorly elucidated and remains a subject of controversy (62).It was described clinically by Wilson in 1869 (42) and histologically by Dubreuil in 1906 (42), It is a dermatosis affecting the stratified squamous epithelium, and can therefore affect the skin, the oral and genital mucosa, the appendages and, more rarely, the conjunctiva and the mucosa of the oesophagus, nose, anus, larynx and bladder (48,46). Disease of the oral mucosa is commonly described in the literature: 50% of subjects with skin lesions have oral lesions, while 25% have only oral lesions. Areas of the oral mucosa can be affected with a certain order of frequency between the different regions (19).

2. Epidemiology

The prevalence of lichen planus is well documented in the literature, It varies from one study to another, but is estimated at 0.9% to 1.2% and no more than 2% in an adult population (35).

Although it affects people of all ages, oral lichen planus is known as a disease of the forties (35). Most studies have found that the average age is between 50 and 55. Oral lichen planus **(OLP)** is rarely diagnosed in children. It has a clear female predilection (36). The 1875 clinical study by Silverman at the University of California San Francisco (53) showed that among 570 patients with LPO, 67% were women with an average age of onset of 52 years. Although approximately 100 familial cases of LPO have been reported in the literature (53), the figures are still low, and these cases can be considered as coincidental, since the disease only affects a maximum of 2% of the population. Oral lichen planus may be isolated or associated with mucosal remnants in :

• 20% of cases are associated with skin disorders

• 15% of cases are associated with genital damage

• 6% of cases are associated with simultaneous damage to 3 other sites:

cutaneous oesophageal genital ophthalmic ....

• On the other hand, 50 to 70% of cutaneous LPs include oral lesions (4).

3. Pathogenesis

The aetiology of LPO remains a controversial subject, and several theories have been put forward.

proposed.

The most likely and best described theory explaining the aetiopathogenesis of LPO is that it was a cell-mediated autoimmune disorder directed against one or more unidentified antigens of the cells of the oral epithelium. The elements supporting this theory are (31):

- The chronicity of the disease,
- Age of onset,
- Preferred gender: female,
- Possible association with other autoimmune diseases and the presence of cytotoxic T cells.

Although the mechanisms of damage are not yet fully understood, two hypotheses dominate:

- An alteration in the keratinocytes, of unknown origin, would lead to the release of antigens and trigger an immune response,
- A reaction by the immune system is thought to be responsible for the alteration and apoptosis of keratinocytes.

Following the 2005 consensus conference, (33) experts assumed that there are several stimuli:

- Viral infection,

- Bacterial molecules,
- Mechanical trauma,
- Systemic therapy
- Sensitive to contact,

These stimulants may activate antigen-presenting cells (APCs) and basal layer keratinocytes, resulting in the synthesis, attraction and stimulation of chemokines, CD8 and CD4 lymphocytes.CD8 lymphocytes are activated by the following antigens:Keratinocytes associated with MHC class 1 (major histocompatibility complex) type 1. Other antigens expressed by keratinocytes and Langerhans cells are associated with MHC class 2 and activate CD4 lymphocytes, followed by various synthetic cytokines (TNF-a, IL-2, IL12, INF-y) which trigger keratinocyte apoptosis.

❖ If the antigens presented by MHC class 1 and 2 are peptides, then the autoimmune nature of LPB would be validated.

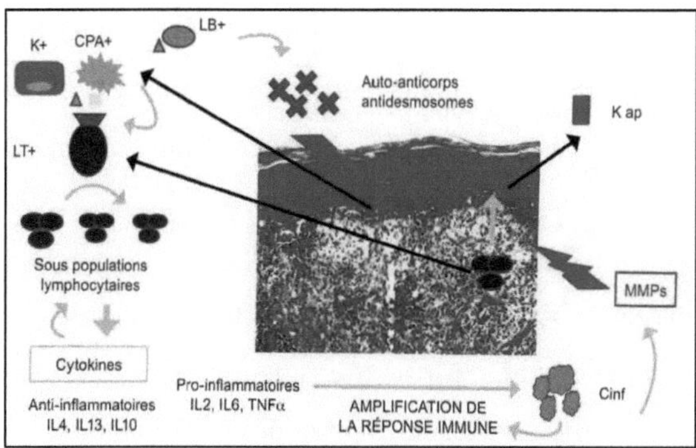

Figure 14: Pathophysiological mechanisms of oral lichen planus (43)

4. Etiology

4.1. Idiopathic lichen planus

Psychological factors are thought to play a role in the pathogenesis of LPO. Patients with OPL have been shown to have higher levels of anxiety, greater depression and increased vulnerability to psychological disorders, compared with healthy controls (54). In addition, LPO exacerbations have been linked to periods of psychological stress and anxiety in some studies. In addition to the chronic discomfort that can lead to stress, LPO patients have been shown to worry about the possibility of malignancy, the contagious nature of the disease.In a study carried out in 2003 by the University of Istanbul,Turkie on 40 LPO patients showed that the levels of anxiety and salivary cortisol measured in a group of LPO patients were statistically correlated and significantly higher than those in a control group (28). Despite the presence of higher levels of psychological stress and anxiety in patients with OPL, the question remains as to whether psychological factors contribute to the aetiology of OPL or whether they are simply driven by the morbidity associated with the condition.

4.2. Lichen planus and associated diseases

Various associations between LPB and certain systemic pathologies are described in the literature. Most are controversial due to the lack of documentation and the existence of regional differences. Some of these associations, such as hypertension, hypothyroidism or diabetes mellitus, may be due to the common age of onset of LPB and these diseases, without any real pathological synergy.

4.2.1. Lichen planus and liver disease

A significantly higher frequency of liver abnormalities is seen in LP patients compared with the normal population (51). In recent years, an increasing number of cases of LP have been reported in association with chronic active hepatitis and primary biliary cirrhosis (primary biliary cholangitis) Korkij et al (14) found an excess of liver abnormalities in LP patients in a control study. Recently, an association between hepatitis C and LPO has been described, although a geographical predilection is suspected. This is the case of the patient in the 2nd clinical observation, whose hepatitis C was detected in association with LPO. Hence the need for further investigations and additional examinations to investigate liver function in any patient presenting with confirmed LPO.

4.2.2. Lichen Plan, Hypertension and diabetes mellitus

An association between LPO, diabetes mellitus and hypertension was first described by Grinspan (2). Although Grinspan syndrome can be observed clinically, the association between the three conditions may simply represent an allergic reaction to drugs used to treat hypertension and/or diabetes rather than a true syndrome.

❖ **Lichen planus and diabetes only**:

The possibility of an association between LPO and diabetes has been fully examined, and the results indicate that such an association is not systematic. The initial reports were due to the fact that the glucose values used at the time to diagnose diabetes were very low compared with today's criteria. In addition, it is possible that the drugs taken by patients to control their diabetes may have induced reactions (35).But this does not prevent the frequency of detection of diabetic patients among LPO patients from being very high, which means that fasting blood glucose tests must be requested in all patients diagnosed with LP. As well as the need to be perfectly prudent when prescribing treatment, especially corticosteroids.

4.2.3. Lichen planus and thyroid disease

The association between OLP and thyroid dysfunction was investigated in a retrospective Finnish study which confirmed a link between OLP and hypothyroidism in particular. This study found that 10% of patients with OLP versus 5% of controls had hypothyroidism; other studies have suggested a relationship between OLP and hyperthyroidism (3).
A thyroid work-up is therefore necessary for LP patients.

4.2.4. Lichen Planus and human papillomavirus (HPV)

Although some studies show that significant human papillomavirus frequency, particularly HPV 16 and 18, in patients with OPL, this association is not well documented. This may be accidental or favoured by an immunosuppressive treatment of oral lichen planus (3).

4.2.5. Inflammatory autoimmune diseases

The literature documents several autoimmune diseases associated with oral lichen planus, including Hashimoto's thyroiditis, Gougerot-Sjogren's syndrome, systemic scleroderma, superficial and deep pemphigus, Good's syndrome (thymoma, vitiligo, alopecia), lupus, lichenoid and atrophic sclerosis, and ulcerative colitis (18).

4.3. Induced lichen planus and lichenoid reactions

Oral contact lichenoid lesions (OCL) are observed in direct topographical relationship with an aggressive agent. This reaction is most often due to dental restoration materials, usually amalgam, or induced by drugs. Once the material or agent in question has been removed and replaced, the majority of cases will be resolved.of these lichenoid lesions disappear within a few months.Contact of the oral mucosa with certain dental restoration materials, in particular mercury-containing amalgams, can cause lesions, and appears to be capable of inducing a sensitivity response leading to immune-mediated damage to the keratinocytes of the basal epithelium. Clinically and histologically, lichenoid lesions can sometimes be indistinguishable from OPL. However, the distinguishing feature is the direct topographical relationship of the lesion to the suspected causative agent. Typical sites are the lateral edges of the tongue and buccal mucosa, sites that have a direct anatomical relationship (i.e. direct contact) with dental restoration(s) or another incriminating contact agent.In PLO lesions, ulcerated areas can also be found in close contact with dental materials. The difference lies in the extent of the lesions. In the case of OLCL, lesions are limited to these contacts, whereas in the case of OLP, lesions may involve sites of the oral mucosa that are not in contact with restorations., gingiva or other mucocutaneous sites, for example the skin or vulvovaginal mucosa (1). The WHO has defined certain conditions for distinguishing between LPO and lesions comparable to LPO.The arguments concerning the necessity and significance of a biopsy for histological confirmation of the diagnosis of lichenoid reaction are not definitive, particularly with regard to the differentiation between PLO and lichenoid reactions (56). A recent study has confirmed the difficulty of distinguishing between the 2 conditions on the basis of histological features alone. Biopsy should be considered when the disease does not present the typical features of the disease (32).

4.4. Graft versus host disease (GVHD)

This condition occurs in patients who have received an allogeneic bone marrow transplant.bone, kidneys... In its acute phase, graft-versus-host disease may manifest as stomatitis and a macular rash of non-specific appearance. In the chronic phase, skin eruptions consisting of lichenoid papules with extensive oral lesions resembling idiopathic LPO are observed. These lesions are known as lichenoid lesions secondary to GVHD (44).

5. Development stages

5.1. The initial phase

The initial phase: lasts 6 to 12 months, with the appearance of white, punctiform, hemispherical lesions, most often in the posterior jugal region; on the back of the tongue, where the keratotic lesions mainly affect the tips of the filiform papillae (Gougerot's papillary lichen). These lesions gradually spread and coalesce to form lines (Wickham's striae), and then form different patterns (reticulated, dendritic, circular LPB, etc.) or keratotic patches. On the back of the tongue, the keratosis invades the entire surface of the papillae and the interpapillary spaces, then very quickly forms an irreversible depapillation on the initial keratotic patches. The keratosis persists and can sometimes take on the appearance of candle wax or sealing bread patches. Apart from the often inconspicuous keratotic patches, damage to the gingival fibromucosa results in the disappearance of its granular appearance and a change in colour to erythema. At this stage, the lesions may regress or disappear with treatment, more rarely spontaneously (36,50).

5.2. The status phase

All these lesions described at the end of the initial phase are similar to those of the state phase, which lasts ten years or more, with a succession of flare-ups and periods of quiescence. Each flare-up is marked by the appearance of erythematous patches, or even erosions, or simply the extension of pre-existing keratotic lesions. Bullae may frequently appear in the posterior jugal region. Functional signs are highly variable: perception of relief or loss of suppleness of the tongue, discomfort, pain or burning sensation in connection with the extent and degree of the flare-up. Outside of flare-ups, there are no symptoms, and LPB takes the form of keratotic lesions which regress over time, but do not completely disappear. The lesions take on a reticulated, dendritic or circinate appearance. However, in patients with dark skin, pigmentation with a black or brown tinge may appear progressively (LPB nigricans), with no clear limit and development favoured by the intensity and frequency of the inflammation.

5.3. The late phase

The late phase begins after several years of evolution, and may occur without the LPB having been diagnosed. It is characterised by the development of an atrophic or scleratrophic state. Atrophy mainly affects the areas of the oral mucosa where there have been active lesions, most often the inner surface of the cheeks. The colour of the mucosa changes and loses its homogeneity: discrete patches of yellowish, brownish or reddish colour are observed; the submucosal capillary network may become transparent due to atrophy. On the back of the tongue, atrophy is seen in the form of stripped patches, which may or may not be covered by a thick keratotic layer. Atrophy of the gingival fibromucosa leads to gingival retraction, often associated with a reduction in the depth of the vestibules, particularly visible in the posterolateral regions. The loss of elasticity of the oral mucosa results in limited mouth opening and reduced tongue protraction.

5.4. Postlichenian stage

The activity of LPO, marked by successive outbreaks, usually wears off eventually. The clinical signs of activity (erythema, erosions, bullae) and the histological signs of activity (lymphocytic infiltrate, exocytosis, hyaline bodies) gradually regress and eventually disappear. Alterations to the mucosa, represented by a variable combination of epithelial atrophy, keratosis, fibrosis of the chorion and possibly pigmentation, are the long-lasting result and the cause of the disease. practically irreversible of past LPO activity. These alterations become clinically apparent when they become significant enough, and persist indefinitely in the oral cavity despite the regression and then disappearance of the Lichenian process. The persistence of these alterations, rare in the skin but common in the oral mucosa, constitutes the post-Lichenian state.

The clinical appearance of the post-Lichenian state is characterised by the almost extinct activity of the LPO, which is very weak or almost non-existent. The only remaining features are: epithelial atrophy (extremely frequent); symmetrical marginal depapillation of the tongue, always respecting the medial posterior area and often the tip.

At this stage, the risk of malignant transformation is high (36).

6. The shapes

6.1. Reticulated form

The reticular form is the most common and is pathognomonic of oral lichen planus, often discovered incidentally. In this form, the lesions are asymptomatic. The primary lesion is a papule, which may be dotted, especially in recent forms, or form a network of white striae. These lesions may also be in the form of dendrites: a fern-leaf appearance, or in the form of rings, circular or confluent in patches, especially in the case of old lichen, or in the form of a sheet, much more common on the dorsal surface of the tongue. This clinical form is generally observed in recent lichen planus or in new flare-ups (60). Clinically, it may appear as a dotted line, a network, dendrites, rings, a circular pattern, a plate or a sheet.

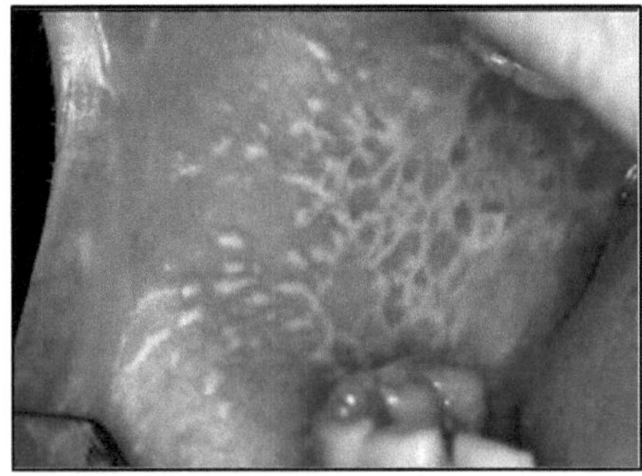

Figure 15: Lichen planus in a network (40).

6.2. Erythematous form

In this form, the erythematous appearance takes centre stage; the blood capillaries are dilated. White lesions are masked, non-existent or reduced to simple mottling by the erythema. Histologically, this is either a recent lichen planus with rather long, frayed ridges, or an active flare-up of an old lichen planus, in which case the ridges tend to be short or even absent. There is an extremely dense lymphocytic infiltrate and numerous lesions of exocytosis. The oral epithelium is thinned but not eroded. This form of lichen is frequently found in vulvovaginal syndrome. This form is not always symptomatic, unlike the erosive and bullous forms (25).

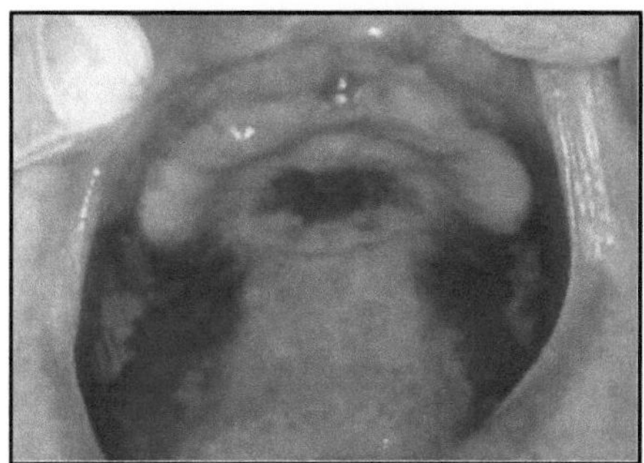

Figure 16: Appearance of Lichen planus erythematosus (25)

6.3. Erosive form

This is the most common form. There are two forms of erosive lichen planus: the minor form and the major form. In both cases, there will be painful erosions of the mucosa ranging from a few millimetres to several centimetres. The erosive oral form is characterised by large, bright red or red varnished, irregular, sometimes angular ulcers, generally symmetrical in appearance and covered with a yellowish fibrinous coating. This erosion reflects focal destruction of the epithelium, which is nibbled away and perforated by the lymphocytic infiltrate, resulting in a fibrino-leukocytic coating. In the minor form, the erosions are quite small and few in number, the white striae are clearly visible and there is an erythema around the periphery. In the major form, erosion predominates, it is sometimes difficult to see the lichen lesions, and the diagnosis is often more difficult to establish. The pain can be violent and burn-like, which makes the diagnosis even more delicate due to the reduced mouth opening. Palpation is painful but no induration can be detected. These pains may be exacerbated by acidic or spicy food, and interfere with oral and dental hygiene, as well as eating in the most extreme cases. This form is highly resistant to treatment and is the most prone to malignant degeneration (2%) **(Figures 17 and 18)** (37).

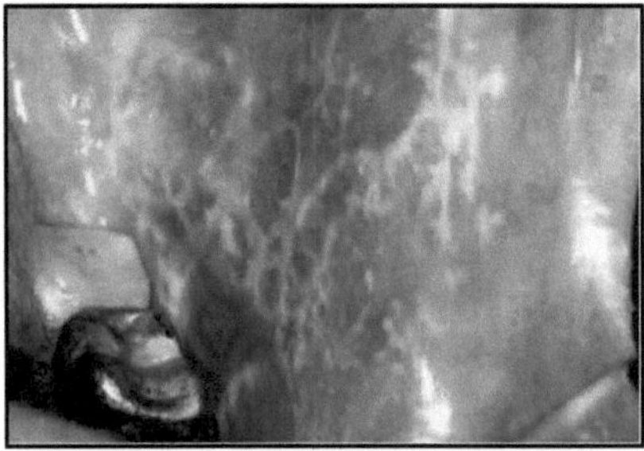

Figure 17: Appearance of minor erosive Lichen planus (37)

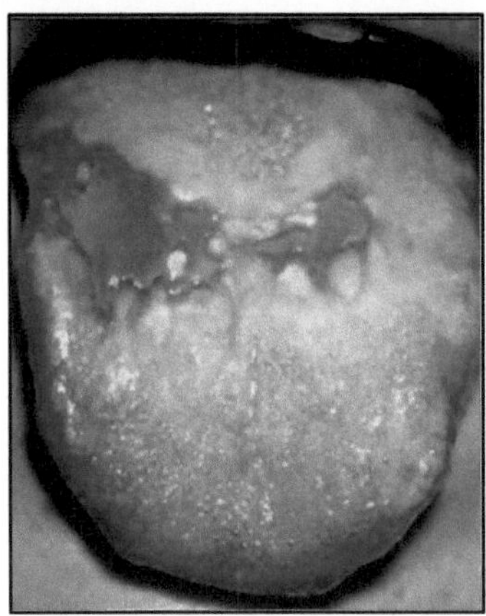

Figure 18: Appearance of major erosive Lichen planus: Erosion and erythema predominate (37)

6.4. Bullous form

Small subepithelial bullae containing a clear or haemorrhagic liquid are found on atrophic and more or less erythematous mucosa. The bullae are rarely intact because they rupture very quickly, so most of the time they cannot be seen and only post-bullous erosions will be seen. There are two types of bullous lichen planus: in the simple form, an often single bulla is present in an area of atrophic lichen planus undergoing a flare-up of inflammation; in the second type of bullous lichen planus, the bullae are multiple and appear at a distance from the lichen areas (**Figure 19**).

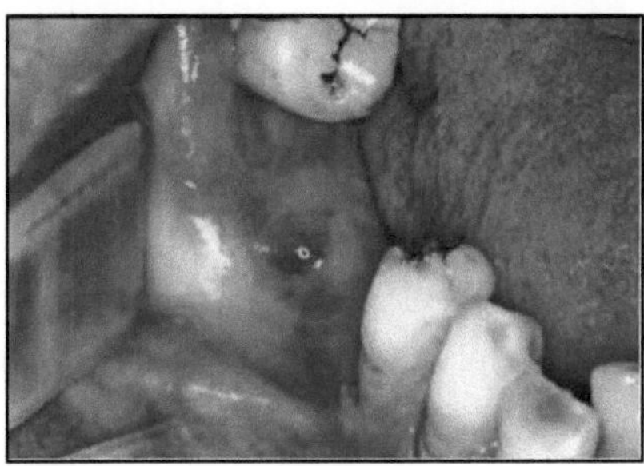

Figure 19: Bullous lichen planus on an area of atrophic and erythematous mucosa (41).

6.5. Atrophic form

This form is the normal evolution of an old LPB that is still active and sometimes undiagnosed, with the development of an atrophic or sclero-atrophic state. The mucosa is shiny or opaline with a smooth appearance, always supple and frequently mixed with other forms, in particular with white streaks around the periphery during periods of activity. The sub-mucosal vascular network is visible by transparency. Involvement is most common in areas where there have been active lesions. The tongue, which is less frequently affected than other mucous membranes, presents marginal, symmetrical and irreversible depapilled patches associated with a more or less thick keratotic layer. A burning sensation on contact with food is common. In the gingival mucosa, there is a loss of "orange peel" staining and atrophy, resulting in a reduction in vestibular depth, mainly in the mandibular molar regions. It also increases the risk of erosions developing from minor trauma. In the most In severe cases, there may be a loss of elasticity associated with limited mouth opening and reduced lingual pro-traction (due to fibrous invasion of the submucosa and superficial muscle fibres). This form is thought to present an increased risk of carcinomatous transformation (23).

6.6. Hypertrophic form

This rare form corresponds to a reactive activitý of epithelial regeneration whose importance exceeds that of the destruction due to lichen activitý. It takes the form of thick, more or less hyperkeratotic lesions, sometimes arranged in islands separated by furrows. Histologically, there is also an appearance of acanthosis and thick, elongated, hyperplastic epithelial ridges with a fairly sparse lymphocytic infiltrate. Superficial hyperkeratosis is often present (30) **(Figure 20).**

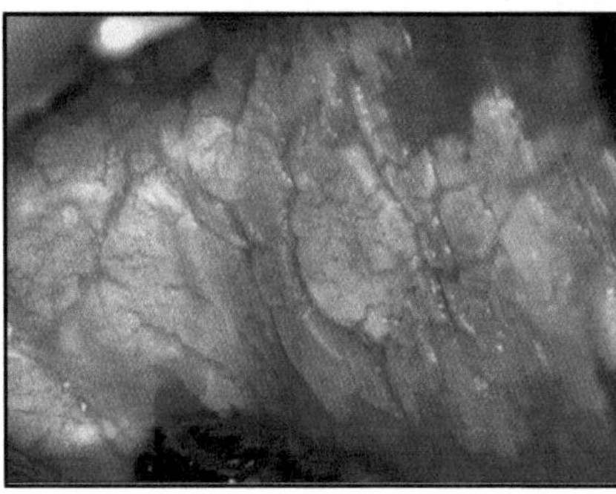

Figure 20: Hypertrophic form of a lichen on the cheek. (According to Kuffer) 2009 (30)

6.7. Pigmented form: LP nigricans

This form is found in dark-skinned individuals. Blackish-brown macules or areoles may appear, associated with white streaks which, in typical cases, gradually take the place of the former white lesions: this is Lichen planus buccalis Nigricans. When these streaks are absent the The differential diagnosis must be made with ethnic pigmentation or smoking-induced melanosis. This form results from the stimulation of melanogenesis by the chronic inflammation present in oral lichen planus. The incontinence of melanin pigment causes melanin pigments to migrate into the superficial chorion as lymphocytes attack the basal layer of the epithelium. These hyperpigmentations occur mainly on the inside of the cheeks and lips, on the tongue and on the soft palate (52).

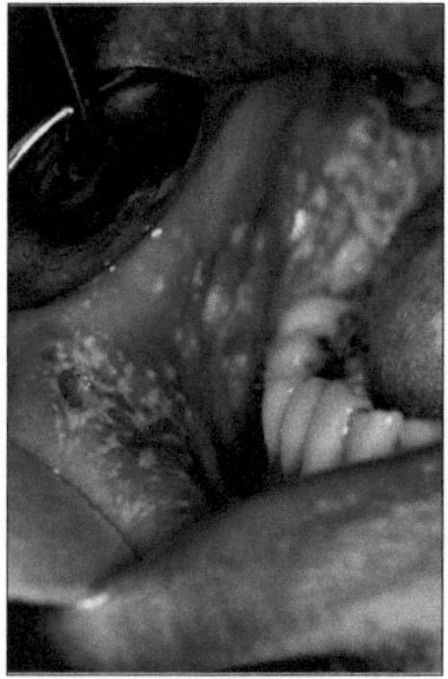

Figure 21: Appearance of lichen planus nigricans on the cheek (61)

7. Evolution, malignant transformation

7.1. Post-Lichenian state

Oral lichen planus develops over a period of years. It differs from that of cutaneous lichen planus, which usually regresses spontaneously. The course can be rapid and debilitating in major erosive forms, but usually The disease progresses very slowly, with successive attacks of varying intensity over many years, or even silently without pain. The disease is often ignored. The evolution of lichen planus into a post-Lichenian state is also explained by the KOEBNER phenomenon (Koebner's phenomenon corresponds, in patients suffering from skin diseases, to the appearance and development of new lesions on healthy skin which has just undergone trauma) because any irritation of a healthy area causes the dermatosis to appear, and similarly, any irritation of an already affected area causes a local exacerbation. In the elderly, lichen activity tends to gradually die out whether or not treatment is given, but damage to the mucosa persists, giving rise to the "irreversible scarring post-lichen condition". The clinical aspect of this post-lichen condition is characterised by :

- Epithelial atrophy is very common.
- Symmetrical marginal depapillation of the tongue and, more rarely, depapillation of the median region.
- Frequent hyperkeratosis.
- Lichenoid streaks of varying thickness, white or opaline, in patches or sheets.
- A more or less smooth surface with a warty appearance.
- Fibrosis with a yellowish mucous membrane of the cheeks
- A reduction in tongue traction or mouth opening.

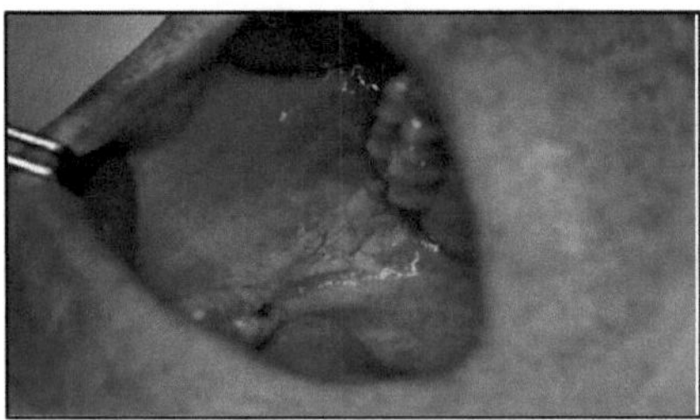

Figure 22: Dr V. Ahossi: Dijon Hospital. Post-lichen condition photo taken at CHU Hôpital général Dijon. (23)

7.2. Malignant transformation: squamous cell carcinoma

Lichen planus is classified as a potentially malignant lesion. The best evidence of the potentially malignant nature of LPO currently available comes from retrospective follow-up and incidence studies. However, there is still considerable controversy regarding the malignant potential of PLO. The frequency of this transformation varies from 0% to 5.8% (7). . The highest rate is found in erythematous and erosive lesions (24). The World Health Organisation has classified LPO as a precancerous condition, which is "a generalised condition associated with a significantly increased risk of cancer" (35). However, the malignant transformation of oral lichen planus leads to differentiated squamous cell carcinoma, which develops progressively, often passing through a verrucous carcinoma stage. The areas affected are those usually affected by lichen planus (inner cheeks, gums, back of the tongue, intermaxillary commissure). Oral squamous cell carcinoma is a serious cancer with a prognosis that is still very poor. These tumours are aggressive, invasive and lymphophilic, and can spread and metastasise (16). It tends to develop on erosive or atrophic lichen planus lesions or post-lichenous lesions and passes through a precursor state of OIN or dysplasia. Degeneration occurs on average within ten years of the diagnosis of oral lichen planus. Squamous cell carcinomas present a wide clinical polymorphism, with the most frequently encountered forms being ulcerative, vegetative and ulcero-vegetative. Other, more atypical forms are sometimes less obvious to diagnose.

8. Positive diagnosis

Confirmation of the diagnosis of oral Lichen planus requires :
Comparison of clinical and histological data: the WHO has proposed the following diagnostic criteria for this lichen, which were modified by van der meij et al 2003.

➤ Modified WHO criteria for the diagnosis of oral lichen planus by Van der meij et al 2003 (58):

• Clinical criteria :

- Bilateral lesions, more or less symmetrical

- Presence of a whitish network (reticulated appearance)

- Bullous or plaque erosive forms are only taken into account.

if there are also reticulated lesions elsewhere in the oral cavity

• Histopathological criteria :

- Presence of a banded inflammatory infiltrate in the superficial part of the chorion, consisting mainly of lymphocytes.
- Liquefaction and degeneration of the basal layer: hyaline balls and colloid bodies: stretcher bodies: homogeneous eosinophilic structures representing apoptotic keratinocytes with nuclear DNA fragmentation
- Absence of epithelial dysplasia (normal maturation of the epithelium, saw-tooth appearance of interpapillary epithelial ridges; abnormal surface keratosis)

- In order to establish a final diagnosis, clinical criteria such as histopathologies must be satisfied!

9. Differential diagnosis

The differential diagnosis of LP depends on the clinical context and the form. The final diagnosis is based on a full medical and dental history, clinical observations, histopathological findings and, if necessary, the results of direct immunofluorescence (DIF).
The differential diagnosis of asymptomatic forms mainly includes various white lesions such as chronic cheek biting, hyperplastic candidiasis and leukoplakia. The bilateral nature and presence of Wickham's striae favour a diagnosis of LP. Biopsy should be considered especially if the clinical context points to a precancerous lesion. However, the differential diagnosis of symptomatic forms

arises with erythematous and bullous lesions such as desquamative gingivitis, mucocutaneous disorders such as mucous membrane pemphigoid, bullous pemphigoid, pemphigus vulgaris, paraneoplastic pemphigus, lupus erythematosus and linear IgA dermatosis. In this context, the biopsy must be accompanied by an IFD test, especially in the absence of Wickham's striae and the presence of a bulla.

Some conditions, such as lichenoid drug and amalgam reactions, graft-versus-host disease and contact stomatitis caused by excessive use of spices, can be difficult to distinguish from LP. Drug-induced lichenoid reactions can occur following the administration of several drugs, such as non-steroidal anti-inflammatory drugs (NSAIDs), certain diuretics, angiotensin-converting enzyme inhibitors, betablockers, penicillamine, allopurinol, chloroquine and many others. These drugs can also exacerbate idiopathic LP. Lichenoid reactions to amalgam are usually unilateral and closely associated with the restoration. They are static, improve with good polishing of the amalgam and regress or disappear completely on removal of the restoration.

Distinguishing between idiopathic LP and lichenoid reactions can be difficult histopathologically and immunologically. The presence of a mixed, deep or perivascular inflammatory infiltrate favours a lichenoid reaction. In its chronic form, graft-versus-host disease can present white reticulated lesions that are clinically similar to LP. The history of a bone marrow transplant is generally sufficient to arrive at a diagnosis. Excessive use of cinnamon can cause lichenoid lesions in the mouth. Depending on the type of product used (toothpaste, mouthwash, chewing gum or sweets), the lesions can be seen on the gums, cheeks or tongue. A full dental history can reveal this The lesions are completely resolved by discontinuing use of the product in question, thereby ruling out LP (26).

9.1. White lesions

Numerous pathologies with more or less frequent white lesions copy the LPB. The most common, in the initial phase, is the confusion between oral candidiasis and the punctiform lesions of the dotted LPB. Tobacco-induced leukoplakia, which is characteristic of smokers, is often accompanied by ectasia of the glandular orifices of the accessory salivary glands, which appear as small, prominent red dots (50).

- Other very rare leukoplakias such as syphilitic leukoplakia (tertiary stage of syphilis) can be found in the lingual area. However, the mucosa is less supple than in LPB.
- Certain reactive keratoses can mimic LPB. They may be endogenous in the vicinity of certain tumours, or of toxic or medicinal origin, leading to the appearance of lichenoid keratotic stomatitis (8). Because of its location, morsicatio buccarum should also be ruled out.
- Proliferative verrucous leukoplakia can mimic the appearance of erosive LPB. Multifocal keratotic lesions form on the gum, tongue and palate, which may progress to erosions (9).
- Chronic discoid lupus erythematosus may mimic or be associated with LPB. The lesions are characterised by a fine keratotic border with radiating white striations. The striations circumscribe a red atrophic or ulcerative plaque interspersed with irregular whitish elements. Lesions occur on the hard palate, buccal mucosa and gingiva.

Skin lesions are generally concomitant.

- Lichenoid keratosis striatum in children and young adults is similar to the appearance of LPB. In the mouth, there are macules and patches of erythema, sometimes with small erosions. The patient also presents with lichenoid papules arranged in parallel striations on the trunk and limbs (29).

In the case of oral localization: diagnoses of keratotic genodermatosis may be evoked:

- Touraine polykeratosis with idiopathic leukoplakia

- Keratotic nevi of the oral mucosa

- Zinsser-Engman-Cole syndrome with similar clinical signs but different histology,

- Kelly-Patterson syndrome with lingual depapillation possibly accompanied by lichenoid white plaque,

- Palmoplantar keratodermas .

9.2. Erythematous and erosive lesions

9.2.1. Pemphigus vulgaris

Pemphigus vulgaris > is an autoimmune bullous intraepithelial dermatosis, which combines erosive and bullous LPB when the striae are barely visible in certain areas. This chronic condition is generally diagnosed by oral erosions, with skin lesions appearing 3 to 6 months after the first oral lesions (57).

Direct immunofluorescence (intercellular deposits in the epithelium, giving a mesh-like appearance) and histological examination (intraepithelial bulla containing acantholytic cells) allow differential diagnosis.Paraneoplastic pemphigus should also be ruled out, as this rare disease bears a strong clinical resemblance to LPB in certain areas.

9.2.2. Bullous pemphigoid

Pemphigoid is a chronic autoimmune bullous dermatosis affecting all mucous membranes (oral, ocular, etc.). The oral form presents with erosive gingivitis more or less associated with bullae and erosions of the palate. Clinical diagnosis is made on the basis of The pincer sign: at the periphery of the gingival erosions, the The epithelium is detached in large, thin flaps at the top of the bullae. The diagnosis of certainty is made following direct immunofluorescence (57). Pemphigoid lichen planus is a rare form of pemphigoid. Developing on a PCL, oral lesions are present in 24% of cases, with gingival and mucosal involvement (9). The clinical appearance is characteristic of LPB: multifocal white streaks are associated with plaques and erosions, or even desquamative gingivitis. The histology is a mixture of LPB and pemphigoid (9).

9.2.3. Erythema multiforme

Seasonal and epidemic, erythema multiforme presents a range of symptoms.

acute mouth ulcers accompanied by fever, similar to LPB. The skin and other mucous membranes may also be affected, presenting characteristic target or cockade lesions.

9.2.4. Chronic ulcerative stomatitis

Chronic ulcerative stomatitis is a rare disease with chronic oral ulceration associated with possible skin involvement. Its clinical and histological aspects are similar to extensive bullous and erosive LPB. If there is any doubt, direct immunofluorescence of the peri-lesional tissue will reveal the presence of immunoglobulin G (IgG) in the basal layers of the epithelium, as well as the presence of stratified epithelium-specific antinuclear antibodies (SES-ANA), the pattern of which is typical of this condition. Resistant to standard LPB treatment, chronic ulcerative stomatitis responds better to treatment with hydroxychloroquine, although relapses are frequent on discontinuation (9).

9.2.5. Atypical mouth ulcers

Further investigations are required

Biology: IFI (antibodies circulating in the blood); serological tests: HIV;
syphilis; HSV
Histology with IFD to detect the cause

10. Treatment

LPB treatment is not curative, but it does help to control symptoms. This symptomatic treatment is extremely important for the patient's quality of life. The therapeutic management of LPB depends on the clinical form. Asymptomatic LPB requires preventive treatment and regular monitoring. On the other hand, treatment of symptomatic LPB allows more effective therapies aimed at eradicating pain and achieving remission. Various treatment modalities have been reported in the literature, most of which are medical, but recent studies have highlighted biological therapies that act on the immune system, as well as other innovations that can reduce the symptoms of LPB.

10.1. Prevention

Before any medicinal treatment, all local aggravating factors should be eliminated, such as poor oral hygiene, ill-fitting dentures, ill-fitting or worn dental restorations, bad habits and tics such as bruxism which traumatise the oral mucosa, as well as tobacco and alcohol which promote and aggravate the development of Lichenian lesions (Koebner's phenomenon) (36).

- **Motivation for oral hygiene**

Optimising oral hygiene is fundamental in the prevention of LPB. Brushing can be difficult to achieve in ulcerative and erosive lesions because of gingival pain and bleeding. Plaque build-up will activate intraoral inflammation and exacerbate LPB activity (22).

Brushing should be carried out at least twice a day, using a soft-bristled toothbrush and mild, fragrance-free toothpaste. Scaling, root planing and professional monitoring should be carried out every 3 to 6 months (45).

- **Elimination of local irritants**

Efforts should be made to minimise mechanical and chemical trauma. A thorough dental examination should be carried out, including an assessment of worn or cracked dental restorations and sharp cusps. The condition of dentures should be assessed, and dentures adjusted or replaced if necessary. Patients should avoid all acidic, spicy, hard and hot foods and drinks. By eliminating exacerbating factors, less severe, reticular and asymptomatic lesions can be maintained or even go into remission. Consumption of alcohol and tobacco, which are known carcinogens, should be reduced, or even eliminated altogether (47,12).

- **Treatment of general illnesses**

It is necessary to treat any illness associated with LPB, or which could aggravate the condition: such as arterial hypertension, diabetes, neoplasia or liver disease.

- **Psychotherapy**

Practitioners should screen patients for depression or anxiety. In a study by Delavarian et al (20), the combination of psychotherapy with the usual treatment for LPB resulted in a significant improvement with a reduction in symptoms compared with the usual treatment for LPB alone. This will make it possible to reduce the use of standard medical treatment.

10.2. Symptomatic treatment

10.2.1. Local corticosteroid therapy

Topical corticosteroids are the drugs most commonly used in the treatment of LPB. 66 to 100% of patients treated respond at least partially to topical corticosteroids, with a variation in efficacy depending on the type and dose of molecule used.Topical corticosteroids can be in the form of cream, gel, bath, etc. mouth or intra-lesional injections. The biggest problem with using topical corticoids in the mouth is the application time: they need to adhere to the buccal mucosa for long enough to do their job. For this reason, they are used in some cases, especially for gingival lichen planus, in combination with an adhesive paste or adhesive tablets (Orobase®), which ensure a longer application time.

Examples of topical corticoids applied to adhesive pastes include triamcinolone acetonide, fluocinolone acetonide, fluocinomide (Topsyne®) and clobetasol propionate (Dermoval®) (49).

10.2.1.1. Prednisolone (solupred®)

The dentist can then prescribe mouthwashes based on Solupred® prednisolone tablets, which are diluted in a glass of water:
- Solupred® effervescent tablets 1 or 2 tablets of 20mg

The mouthwash should be left on for two to three minutes without rinsing before being used.spit out, and is carried out two or three times a day. In the same way, it will be necessary to reduce doses gradually before stopping mouthwash...(27)

10.2.1.2. Clobetasone propionate (Dermoval®)

Clobetasol proprionate appears to be the most effective topical corticosteroid,

This corticosteroid is more effective in an adhesive paste than on its own. Clobetasol propionate should therefore be used with Orobase® (mixed in equal quantities), and applied twice a day (15).

10.2.1.3. Betamethasone (Diprosone®)

Especially in association of several corticoids including βmethasone (Diprosone®),proprionate clobetasol (Dermoval®), and fluocinonide (Topsyne®) is indicated particularly in cases of gum disease resistant to topical and systemic treatment. This preparation is applied in the evening at bedtime. It can be inserted into a moulded polyurethane mouthpiece. Treatment is tapered over several months (from one to three months).to prevent recurrences.
However, attention must be paid to the undesirable effects of local corticoids, such as viral, fungal, parasitic and bacterial infections. This is why an antifungal agent is sometimes added to increase the effectiveness of the treatment (1).

10.2.1.4. Triancinolone(kenacort retard®)

Used mainly as an intralesional treatment in cases of resistance to other oral treatments; its effect is longer-lasting.

10.2.2. Systemic corticosteroid therapy

Systemic corticosteroid therapy may be indicated, alone or in combination with local treatment, especially in severe, disabling, extensive and bulloerosive forms in flare-up. In the absence of contraindication, prednisone (Cortancyl®) is prescribed at a dose of 1 mg/kg per day for ten to 15 days, then rapidly tapered over one to two months, followed by local corticosteroids to prevent relapses on discontinuation. A comparison of local corticosteroids (Dermoval® in Orabase® twice daily) and systemic corticosteroids (Solupred 50 mg/d) in LPBE relapses was studied in 49 patients (6): no significant difference was noted in the efficacy of the two treatments, but the side effects were much greater in the prednisolone group.Regular monitoring is recommended, particularly during corticosteroid therapy. Systemic: oral candidiasis remains the most frequent complication. However, the of treatments antifungal treatments should not be systematic.

10.2.3. Retinoids

Retinoids act on the proliferation and differentiation of keratinocytes and have an anti-inflammatory and immunomodulatory effect. Topical retinoids are the second line of treatment, and have been shown to be effective in atrophic or erosive forms of LPB (49).

10.2.3.1. Topical retinoids

Topical retinoids have shown definite efficacy in several studies. **Isotretinoin** proved effective in two randomised studies: the difference was significant at two months, despite burning and irritation, with a recrudescence of sensations pain and an increase in sensitivity to hot and spicy foods, described by patients as transient and acceptable after the first few applications. The alcoholic excipients used cause immediate burning sensations on application and episodes of dryness.Another study compared the efficacy of two concentrations of the active ingredient, 0.05 and 0.18%, applied twice daily. The results with the 0.18% preparation were better in atrophic and erosive forms, as well as in dysplastic phenomena starting with histological confirmation (21). Tretinoin (all-trans-retinoic acid), applied locally twice a day for four months, led to a significant improvement (94% vs. 21% with placebo) in LPBE lesions, with side effects such as minimal burning.Tazarotene gel 0.1% applied twice a day for eight weeks improved LPB lesions, particularly hyperkeratotic forms (17).

10.2.3.2. Systemic retinoids

Vitamin A is known to be effective in regulating the proliferation and differentiation of the epithelium, and its deficiency can lead to hyperkeratosis of the skin and squamous metaplasia of the mucous membranes. Systemic retinoids have therefore been reported in the treatment of symptomatic lichen planus, particularly LPBE.

10.2.4. Calcineurin inhibitors

10.2.4.1. Cyclosporin A

Cyclosporine A (Sandimmun®, Neoral®) has immunosuppressive properties through its modulatory action on T lymphocytes (inhibition of IL-2 production) and the synthesis of pro-inflammatory cytokines, which explains its properties in immunological processes, particularly autoimmune processes such as in LP. It is used as a second-line treatment in topical form: its efficacy, although recognised in current practice, is debated due to the lack of randomised controlled trials.
Cyclosporine is most often used as a mouthwash, or applied with a finger in a

conventional oily solution. Some patients prefer to use cyclosporine extracted from capsules, which is more viscous and better suited to erosion than solution (6).

10.2.4.2. Topical tacrolimus (Protopic®)

Tacrolimus is an immunosuppressive macrolide with a mechanism of action similar to that of cyclosporine. Its main advantage over cyclosporine lies in its hydrophobic properties and its ability to be absorbed adequately through the epithelium, both in healthy and damaged mucosa. The use of topical tacrolimus, as a mouthwash or 0.1% cream (55), applied two to four times a day, results in rapid improvement in symptoms, in an average of two weeks, and at least partial healing of ulcerations of the oral mucosa in patients resistant to local corticosteroids or systemic treatments. This treatment has shown definite efficacy, with an improvement in LPBE symptoms, particularly pain, as early as the second week. This treatment is only suspensive, with lesions recurring on average two months after applications are stopped. Side effects are minor but frequent, such as a burning sensation or local irritation, observed in 30% of cases. Pigmentation of the buccal mucosa appeared under tacrolimus treatment and regressed spontaneously after applications were stopped (39).

10.2.5. Other cortisone-sparing treatments

10.2.5.1. Hydroxychloroquine (Plaquenil®)

Synthetic antimalarials, in particular hydroxychloroquine (Plaquenil®), have multiple therapeutic properties which are thought to be linked to the inhibition of effector mechanisms of inflammation and immunomodulation based on the inhibition of antigen presentation to T cells.Hydroxychloroquine has proven its value in the management of autoimmune diseases such as rheumatoid arthritis and lupus erythematosus. Hydroxychloroquine, in doses of 200 to 400 mg a day, has also proved effective for LPO. However, this was an open trial involving only 30 patients.What's more, it's not always effective and it can take several months to improve.Hydroxychloroquine is not a completely harmless drug. Before starting treatment, a basic visual acuity test should be carried out and repeated every 6 to 12 months to check for ocular toxicity. Lichenoid skin reactions triggered by UV light (sunlight) have also been reported with this drug.As well as haematological abnormalities and disturbances in liver function tests. Therefore, regular complete blood counts and liver function tests are warranted. Pre-existing retinopathy, psoriasis and porphyria are known contraindications to the use of hydroxychloroquine (14,13).

10.2.5.2. Systemic immunosuppressants

Azathioprine (Imurel) has been reported to be successful as a "cortisone-sparing agent" for cutaneous lichen planus, and there are few published studies suggesting that it may play a similar role in OPL. In general, the initial dose should be approximately 1.0 mg/kg/d (50 to 100 mg), increased progressively in increments of 0.5 mg/kg/d over several weeks, if necessary up to a maximum dose of 2 mg/kg/d. If the patient does not improve within 3 months, azathioprine should be discontinued (34).

10.2.5.3. Phototherapy

PUVA therapy has been reported in several studies in the treatment of LP in its pure cutaneous or mixed cutaneous-mucosal form.However, side effects were noted. The oncological risk associated with the risk of malignant transformation of LPB makes this therapeutic combination a delicate one. The significant carcinological risk contraindicates PUVA therapy in the treatment of LPB (59).

10.2.6.Other treatments under study

Numerous therapies have been studied, with varying degrees of effectiveness:

- Tetracycline mouthwash has been tried effectively in one case of relapsing

LPB.

• Doxycycline can be used in a few reported cases of gingival lesions, but is of little use in other areas.

• Griseofulvin, 500 mg/d for two to six months, is of minor benefit, with recurrence on discontinuation of treatment. A recent study involved a group of patients with LP treated with griseofulvin, 6 of whom had LPBE. For these erosive oral lesions, a favourable clinical response was obtained in 66% of cases (5).

10.2.7.Surgery

Some authors have previously described the management of LP by surgery exeresis.

10.2.8.Oral lichen planus and laser

In recent years, phototherapy (lasers, UV therapy and photodynamic therapy) seems to be an interesting new approach that can be successfully applied in the treatment of PLO. The word LASER is short for "Light Amplification by Stimulated Emission of Radiation". There are two main groups of laser therapy: laser ablation (vaporisation) and laser biomodulation, and both are well documented in the treatment of low-level laser therapy (LLLT).

The primary outcome associated with the use of the diode laser in the treatment of OPL was symptom (pain) relief. All the included studies on the use of diode laser with the exception of the study by Cafaro et al. used the Visual Analogue Scale (VAS), a reliable non-verbal scale to assess pain levels. All these studies concluded that LLLT was effective in reducing the pain associated with oral lichen planus.However, the main disadvantage of laser surgery as a treatment modality is tissue destruction, resulting in limited histopathological analysis. Despite the effectiveness of the laser as a new approach that can be successfully applied in the treatment of cortico-resistant and pain-prone patients, the cost of laser equipment and the need for laser-qualified personnel with specialist knowledge and experience limit dentists' access to these advantages of the laser. The second limitation is the follow-up period, as several studies had a short follow-up period or did not clearly indicate the duration of follow-up. A longer follow-up period might have produced different results.In order to determine the most effective way of using laser therapy for the elimination of LPB (optimal wavelength, energy, duration and frequency of treatment), further well-designed clinical studies with precise laser parameters, a large number of patients and prolonged, long-term follow-up are required (10).

10.2.9. Oral lichen planus and fibrin-rich plasma (FRP) Although

FRP injections are not a standard treatment option, they have been shown to be equally effective in reducing the symptoms and size of LPB lesions. The results obtained with FRP are similar to those obtained with TA: triamcinolone acetonide. Further data needs to be collected on the durability of the conditions in a longer follow-up with more samples. In conclusion, given the separate mouth study design and the lack of data on the possible systemic effects of TA injections, there is a need to clarify the true efficacy of PLO treatment with i-PRF and the dose to be used. The results described are promising, but future research is needed to determine whether APCs could be an alternative to corticosteroids in topical therapy for OLP, thanks to the lower biological and economic costs incurred by patients and to the lower impact on the healthcare system (9).

10.2.10. Oral lichen planus and platelet-rich plasma (PRP)

Platelet-rich plasma (PRP) is a concentration of human platelets three to five times higher than the physiological concentration of thrombocytes in whole blood.This product is characterised by large quantities of growth factors, which are released after platelet activation and are capable of stimulating the production of extracellular matrix collagen. In dentistry and maxillofacial surgery, the use of PRP has been described, for example, in the treatment of bone diseases such as medication-related osteonecrosis of the jaws, particularly as a complement to the surgical protocol, in the form of a gel for topical application.A recent clinical study in Italy, 2018 has shown that PRP has proven almost equivalent efficacy to corticosteroids in the management of potentially malignant erosive LPB. Thanks to its anti-inflammatory effects, wound healing stimulation properties and biological safety, PRP could be used as a new alternative therapy in the treatment of oral lichen planus. It is clear that more detailed prospective studies on a larger group of patients and with a longer follow-up period are necessary (38).

CONCLUSION

Oral lichen planus remains a benign chronic pathology commonly seen in the routine practice of specialists in oral medicine and surgery and dentists in general practice. Its etiopathogenesis is still poorly defined and multifactorial.Its clinical diagnosis is sometimes very obvious, but confirmation requires the combination of clinical and histopathological data.These diagnostic criteria must be well known by any dentist in order to be able to refer or manage these patients and not confuse them with the other pathologies of the oral mucosa, which are multiple, whether in the symptomatic or asymptomatic phase.The management of this dermatosis requires a preventive phase aimed at restoring the oral cavity and eliminating irritants. Any associated pathology detected must be well explored and treated Subsequently, it is necessary to manage the symptoms in the activity phase by the different therapies proposed. The quiescence phase requires a simple check to avoid the reactivation of symptoms. Although it is a chronic and benign condition, oral lichen planus requires careful and continuous monitoring for fear of the risk of malignant transformation, hence the role of the dentist in motivating and monitoring patients.

REFERENCES

1. Al-Hashimi I, Schifter M, Lockhart PB et al.

Oral lichen planus and oral lichenoid lesions: Diagnostic and therapeutic considerations. Oral Surg Oral Med Oral Pathol Oral Radiol Endod 2007;103:1-12.

2. Aljabre SH.

Grinspan's syndrome.J Am Acad Dermatol 1994;30(4):671.

3. Alrashdan MS, Cirillo N, McCullough M.

Oral lichen planus: A literature review and update. Arch Dermatol Res 2016;308(8):539-51.

4. Andreasen JO.

Oral lichen planus: I. A clinical evaluation of 115 cases. Oral Surg Oral Med Oral Pathol 1968;25(1):31-42.

5. Carbone M, Conrotto D, Carrozzo M, Broccoletti R, Gandolfo S, Scully C.

Topical corticosteroids in association with miconazole and chlorhexidine in the long-term management of atrophic-erosive oral lichen planus: A placebo-controlled and comparative study between clobetasol and fluocinonide.
Oral Dis 1999;5(1):44-9.

6. Carbone M, Goss E, Carrozzo M et al.

Systemic and topical corticosteroid treatment of oral lichen planus: a comparative study with long-term follow-up: Corticosteroid treatment of oral lichen planus.J Oral Pathol Med 2003;32(6):323-9.

7. Cardozo Pereira AL, Castro Jacques M, Cabral MG, Cardoso AS, Ramos-e-Silva M.
Oral lichen planus part II: Therapy and malignant transformation. Skinmed 2004;3(1):19-22.

8. Cendras J, Bonnetblanc JM.

Erosive oral lichen planus .Ann Dermatol Venereol 2009;136(5):458-70.

9. Cheng YS, Gould A, Kurago Z, Fantasia J, Muller S. Diagnosis of oral lichen planus: A position paper of the American academy of oral and maxillofacial pathology.Oral Surg Oral Med Oral Pathol Oral Radiol 2016;122(3):332-54.

10. Dammak N, Slim A, Hmaissi C et al.

Efficacy of laser in the treatment of oral lichen planus: A systematic review. Actual Tunis Odontol 2020;10(1):76-85.

11. Dey VK.

Netherton syndrome: A rare genodermatosis.Indian Dermatol Online J 2011;2(1):38-9.

12. Eisen D, Carrozzo M, Bagan Sebastian JV, Thongprasom K. Number V oral lichen planus: Clinical features and management. Oral Dis 2005;11(6):338-49.

13. Eisen D.

Hydroxychloroquine sulfate (Plaquenil) improves oral lichen planus: An open trial.J Am Acad Dermatol 1993;28(4):609-12.

14. Eisen D.

The clinical manifestations and treatment of oral lichen planus.Dermatol Clin 2003;21(1):79-89.

15. García-Pola MJ, González-Álvarez L, Garcia-Martin JM.

Treatment of oral lichen planus. Systematic review and therapeutic guide.

Med Clin 2017;149(8):351-62.

16. Gaultier F.

Squamous cell carcinoma and mouth ulcers. Réal Clin 2016;2:83-90.

17. Giustina TA, Stewart JC, Ellis CN et al.

Topical application of isotretinoin gel improves oral lichen planus. A double-blind study. Arch Dermatol 1986;122(5):534-6.

18. Gururaj N, Hasinidevi P, Janani V, Divynadaniel T. Diagnosis and management of oral lichen planus-Review. J Oral Maxillofac Pathol 2021;25(3):383.

19. Hamour AF, Klieb H, Eskander A.

Oral lichen planus.

CMAJ 2020;192(31):E892.

20. Hampf BG, Malmström MJ, Aalberg VA, Hannula JA, Vikkula J.

Psychiatric disturbance in patients with oral lichen planus. Oral Surg Oral Med Oral Pathol 1987;63(4):429-32.

21. Hersle K, Mobacken H, Sloberg K, Thilander H.

Severe oral lichen planus: Treatment with an aromatic retinoid (etretinate). Br J Dermatol 1982;106(1):77-80.

22. Holmstrup P, Schiøtz AW, Westergaard J.

Effect of dental plaque control on gingival lichen planus.Oral Surg Oral Med Oral Pathol 1990;69(5):585-90.

23. Ismail SB, Kumar SKS, Zain RB.

Oral lichen planus and lichenoid reactions: Etiopathogenesis, diagnosis, management and malignant transformation.
J Oral Sci 2007;49(2):89-106.

24. Jaafari-Ashkavandi Z, Mardani M, Pardis S, Amanpour S.

Oral mucocutaneous diseases: Clinicopathologic analysis and malignant transformation.
J Craniofac Surg 2011;22(3):949-51.

25. Jindal R, De D, Kanwar AJ.

Bullous oral lichen planus: An unusual variant.

Indian Dermatol Online J 2011;2(1):39-40.

26. Kauzman A, Cox M, Tran JB, Lalonde B.

Oral lichen planus - update and review of the literature.

J Ordre Dent Québec 2006;43:153-61.

27. Kellett JK, Ead RD.

Treatment of lichen planus with a short course of oral prednisolone.

Br J Dermatol 2006;123(4):550-1.

28. Koray M, Dülger O, Horasanli S et al.

The evaluation of anxiety and salivary cortisol levels in patients with oral lichen planus. Oral Dis 2003;9(6):298-301.

29. Kuffer R, Lombardi T, Husson-Bui C et al.

Oral lichen planus. In: Kuffer R, Lombardi T, Husson-Bui C et al, eds. La muqueuse buccale de la clinique au traitement.
Paris: Med'com, 2009:77-89.

30. Kuffer R.

The oral mucosa: from clinic to treatment.

Paris: Éditions Med'com, 2009.

31. Kurago ZB.

Etiology and pathogenesis of oral lichen planus: An overview.

Oral Surg Oral Med Oral Pathol Oral Radiol 2016;122(1):72-80.

32. Larsson Å, Warfvinge G.

Oral lichenoid contact reactions may occasionally transform into malignancy.
Eur J Cancer Prev 2005;14(6):525-9.

33. Lodi G, Scully C, Carrozzo M, Griffiths M, Sugerman PB, Thongprasom K.

Current controversies in oral lichen planus: Report of an international consensus meeting. Part 1. Viral infections and etiopathogenesis.
Oral Surg Oral Med Oral Pathol Oral Radiol Endod 2005;100(1):40-51.

34. Lozada F.

Prednisone and azathioprine in the treatment of patients with vesiculoerosive oral diseases.
Oral Surg Oral Med Oral Pathol 1981;52(3):257-60.

35. Lozada-Nur F, Miranda C.

Oral lichen planus: Epidemiology, clinical characteristics, and associated diseases.
Semin Cutan Med Surg 1997;16(4):273-7.

36. Lysitsa S, Abi Najm S, Lombardi T, Samson J.

Oral lichen planus: Natural history of a malignant transformation.

Med buccale Chir buccale 2007;13(1):19-29.

37. Mauskar M.

Erosive Lichen Planus.

Obstet Gynecol Clin North Am 2017;44(3):407-20.

38. Merigo E, Oppici A, Parlatore A et al.

Platelet-rich plasma (PRP) rinses for the treatment of non-responding oral lichen planus: A case report.
Biomedicines 2018;6(1):1-4.

39. Olivier V, Lacour JP, Mousnier A, Garraffo R, Monteil RA, Ortonne JP.

Treatment of chronic erosive oral lichen planus with low concentrations of topical tacrolimus: An open prospective study.
Arch Dermatol 2002;138(10):1335-8.

40. Orme CM, Kim RH, Brinster N, Elbuluk N, Franks AG.

Lichen planus pigmentosus.

Dermatol Online J 2016;22(12):17-9.

41. Papara C, Danescu S, Sitaru C, Baican A.

Challenges and pitfalls between lichen planus pemphigoides and bullous lichen planus.
Australas J Dermatol 2022;63(2):165-71.

42. Parashar P.

Oral lichen planus.

Otolaryngol Clin North Am 2011;44(1):89-107.

43. Payeras MR, Cherubini K, Figueiredo MA, Salum FG.

Oral lichen planus: Focus on etiopathogenesis.

Arch Oral Biol 2013;58(9):1057-69.

44. Ramachandran V, Kolli SS, Strowd LC. Review of graft-versus-host disease. Dermatol Clin 2019;37(4):569-82.

45. Ramón-Fluixá C, Bagán-Sebastián J, Milián-Masanet M, Scully C. Periodontal status in patients with oral lichen planus: A study of 90 cases. Oral Dis 1999;5(4):303-6.

46. Roopashree MR, Gondhalekar RV, Shashikanth MC, George J, Thippeswamy SH, Shukla A.

Pathogenesis of oral lichen planus - a review.

J Oral Pathol Med 2010;39(10):729-34.

47. Schlosser BJ.

Lichen planus and lichenoid reactions of the oral mucosa.

Dermatol Ther 2010;23(3):251-67.

48. Scully C, Carrozzo M.

Oral mucosal disease: Lichen planus.

Br J Oral Maxillofac Surg 2008;46(1):15-21.

49. Scully C, Eisen D, Carrozzo M.

Management of oral lichen planus.

Am J Clin Dermatol 2000;1(5):287-306.

50. Seintou A, Gaydarov N, Lombardi T, Samson J.

Natural history and malignant transformation of oral lichen planus. Part 1: Mice in focus.Med Buccale Chir Buccale 2012;18(2):89-107.

51. Shai A, Halevy S.

Lichen planus and lichen planus-like eruptions: Pathogenesis and associated diseases.Int J Dermatol 1992;31(6):379-84.

52. Shklar G, McCarthy PL.

The oral lesions of lichen planus: Observations on 100 cases.

Oral Surg Oral Med Oral Pathol 1961;14(2):164-81.

53. Silverman S Jr, Gorsky M, Lozada-Nur F.

A prospective follow-up study of 570 patients with oral lichen planus: Persistence, remission, and malignant association.
Oral Surg Oral Med Oral Pathol 1985;60(1):30-4.

54. Soto Araya M, Rojas Alcayaga G, Esguep A.

Asociación entre alteraciones psicológicas y la presencia de Liquen plano oral, Síndrome boca urente y Estomatitis aftosa recividante.
Med Oral Patol Oral Cir Bucal 2004;9(1):1-7.

55. Swift JC, Rees TD, Plemons JM, Hallmon WW, Wright JC.

The effectiveness of 1% pimecrolimus cream in the treatment of oral erosive lichen planus.
J Periodontol 2005;76(4):627-35.

56. Thornhill MH, Sankar V, Xu XJ et al.

The role of histopathological characteristics in distinguishing amalgam-associated oral lichenoid reactions and oral lichen planus.
J Oral Pathol Med 2006;35(4):233-40.

57. Vaillant L, Goga D. Dermatologie buccale. Paris: Doin Editions, 1998.
58. Van der Meij EH, Mast H, Van der Waal I.

The possible premalignant character of oral lichen planus and oral lichenoid lesions: A prospective five-year follow-up study of 192 patients. Oral Oncol

2007;43(8):742-8.

59. Wolff D, Anders V, Corio R et al.

Oral PUVA and topical steroids for treatment of oral manifestations of chronic graft-vs.-host disease. Photodermatol Photoimmunol Photomed 2004;20(4):184-90.

Internet references

60. Benyahya I, Bouzoubaa S.

Oral lichen planus: an update [Online].[Accessed on 12/01/2023], available from the URL: https://pesquisa.bvsalud.org/portal/resource/pt/afr-197697

61. Oral dermatology.

Pigmented lesions [Online].[Accessed 12/01/2023], available from the URL: https://www.dermato-buccale.com/lesions-pigmentees/lichen- nigricans.htm

62. Santé Magazine.

Lichen planus: everything you need to know about this chronic inflammatory skin disease [Online].[Accessed on 12/01/2023], available from the URL: https://www.santemagazine.fr/sante/fiche-maladie/lichen-plan-177633

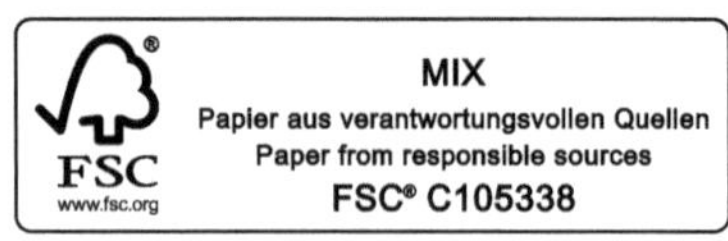

Printed by Books on Demand GmbH, Norderstedt / Germany